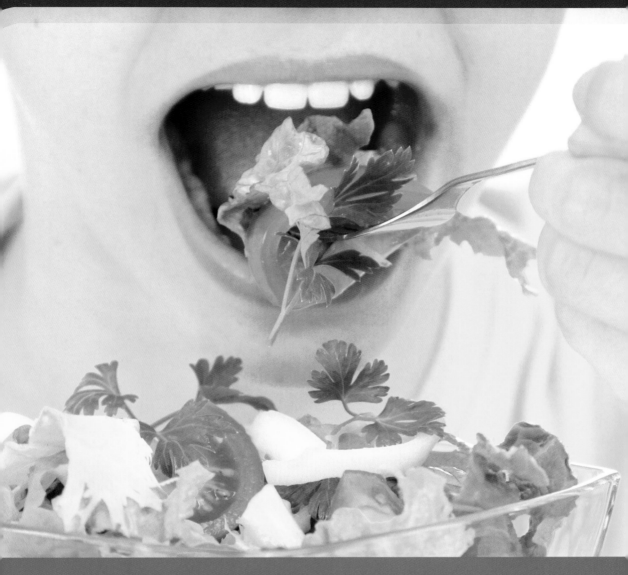

NUTRITION MYTHS,
BUSTED!

by Marne Ventura

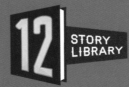

12 STORY LIBRARY

www.12StoryLibrary.com

12-Story Library is an imprint of Peterson Publishing Company and Press Room Editions.

Produced for 12-Story Library by Red Line Editorial

Photographs ©: kokanphoto/Shutterstock Images, cover, 1, 23; FSA/OWI Collection/Library of Congress, 4; Monkey Business Images/Shutterstock Images, 5, 17, 21, 29; Wutthichai/Shutterstock Images, 6; k r e f/Shutterstock Images, 7; George Dolgikh/Shutterstock Images, 8; Russell Lee/FSA/OWI Collection/Library of Congress, 9; Marty Lederhandler/AP Images, 10; Olesya Feketa/Shutterstock Images, 11; Lesya Dolyuk/Shutterstock Images, 12; Marcos Mesa Sam Wordley/Shutterstock Images, 13, 28; res-art/iStockphoto, 15; kazoka/Shutterstock Images, 16; Plustwentyseven/DigitalVision/Thinkstock, 18; p.studio66/Shutterstock Images, 19; Syda Productions/Shutterstock Images, 20; Aaron Amat/Shutterstock Images, 22; Cherry-Merry/Shutterstock Images, 24; OcusFocus/iStockphoto, 25; Fuse/Thinkstock, 26; Gts/Shutterstock Images, 27

Library of Congress Cataloging-in-Publication Data
Names: Ventura, Marne, author.
Title: Nutrition myths, busted! / by Marne Ventura.
Description: North Mankato, MN : 12-Story Library, [2017] | Series: Science
   myths, busted! | Audience: Grades 4 to 6. | Includes bibliographical
   references and index.
Identifiers: LCCN 2016002365 (print) | LCCN 2016004731 (ebook) | ISBN
   9781632353047 (library bound : alk. paper) | ISBN 9781632353542 (pbk. :
   alk. paper) | ISBN 9781621434696 (hosted ebook)
Subjects: LCSH: Nutrition--Miscellanea--Juvenile literature. |
   Dietetics--Miscellanea--Juvenile literature.
Classification: LCC TX355 .V437 2017 (print) | LCC TX355 (ebook) | DDC
   613.202--dc23
LC record available at http://lccn.loc.gov/2016002365

Printed in the United States of America
Mankato, MN
May, 2016

Access free, up-to-date content on this topic plus a full digital version of this book. Scan the QR code on page 31 or use your school's login at 12StoryLibrary.com.

Table of Contents

Busted: Carrots Help You See in the Dark

During World War II (1939–1945), the German military repeatedly bombed the United Kingdom. Most German bombing raids happened at night. The British used radar to detect German bombers. But they did not want the Germans to know about their technology. Instead, the British military claimed pilots were eating lots of carrots.

The carrots allowed pilots to see in the dark, the British said. Many people believed the military. Carrots earned the reputation for helping people see in the dark.

As early as 490 BCE, people believed diet and eyesight were connected. It took nearly 1,000 years to learn how. Ancient Greek thinker Hippocrates studied night

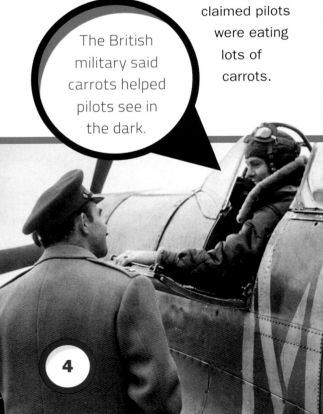

The British military said carrots helped pilots see in the dark.

9,189
International units of vitamin A in 0.5 cup (227 g) of raw carrots.

- The British military said pilots ate carrots to improve their night vision.
- Vitamins were discovered in foods in the early 1900s.
- Vitamin A is used to make retinal, which helps people see in dim light.

blindness. People with night blindness cannot see in dim light. Hippocrates thought eating raw liver could cure it. Eating liver seemed to make night blindness go away. Until the twentieth century, nobody understood why.

In the early 1900s, scientists studied the chemicals in foods. Researchers suspected food contained unidentified nutrients. In 1912, biochemist Casmir Funk identified substances in food. He called them *vital amines*. The substances were later called vitamins. Liver contains lots of vitamin A. The vitamin A in liver and other foods cures night blindness.

A half-cup of carrots gives you enough vitamin A for the day.

GEORGE WALD

In 1932, New York doctor George Wald dissected 300 frog eyes. He tested them to learn about the chemicals inside. He discovered the part of the eye called the retina contains vitamin A. He confirmed a lack of vitamin A causes night blindness.

Carrots contain beta carotene, a nutrient the body turns into vitamin A. Your eyes need vitamin A to make retinal. Retinal is a chemical. It allows people to see in dim light. Without getting enough beta carotene, people might have trouble seeing in dim light. But no amount of carrots will make human eyes see in total darkness. Eating carrots does not improve other eye problems, either.

5

Busted: Vitamin C Prevents Colds

By the time he won the Nobel Peace Prize in 1962, Linus Pauling was a respected scientist. He had also won the Nobel Prize in chemistry eight years prior. His work in chemistry led him to study vitamins. He wanted to discover if vitamin C prevented colds.

In 1970, people trusted the famous scientist's advice. Pauling conducted a study with schoolchildren in Switzerland. He concluded that taking a vitamin C pill prevents and lessens cold symptoms. Millions of people have

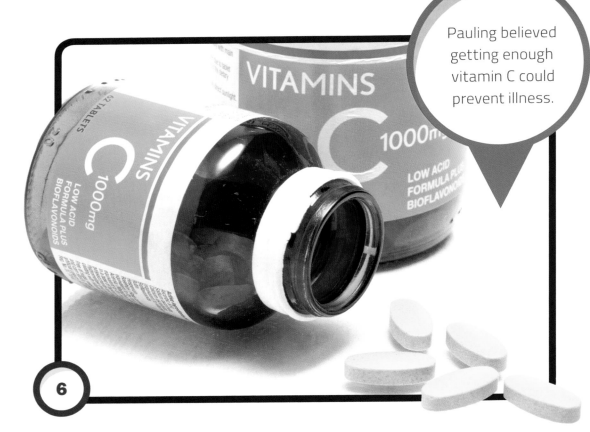

Pauling believed getting enough vitamin C could prevent illness.

VITAMINS C 1000mg LOW ACID FORMULA PLUS BIOFLAVONOIDS

followed Dr. Pauling's advice.

Other scientists tried to find the same evidence. They conducted studies in the United States, Canada, and the Netherlands. None of the studies backed up Pauling's findings. They did find evidence that eating more produce helps people stay healthy. Fruits and vegetables are high in vitamin C. But further research fails to show they prevent the common cold.

Lemons, limes, and oranges help prevent scurvy.

100
Percent of fruits and vegetables that contain vitamin C.

- Pauling won the Nobel Prize in chemistry in 1954 and the Nobel Peace Prize in 1962.
- In 1970, Pauling found colds could be prevented with vitamin C pills.
- Since 1970, scientists have failed to confirm his findings.

SCURVY

Before canned and frozen foods were invented, sailors got a disease called scurvy. Many sailors on long voyages often got the disease. They ate only dried meat and bread and got sick or died. But sailors who ate citrus fruits stayed healthy. People knew that eating citrus fruits helped keep scurvy at bay. But for hundreds of years, they did not know why. In the 1930s, scientists discovered the vitamin C in citrus fruits prevents scurvy.

Busted: White and Whole-Grain Bread Are Equally Nutritious

Both white and whole-grain breads are made from wheat. But they are made in different ways. People used to think white and whole-grain bread just looked different. But it turns out one is more nutritious than the other.

Grains of wheat have three parts. The bran and germ contain fiber, B vitamins,

Whole-grain bread contains more nutrition than white bread does.

protein, minerals, and healthy fats. The endosperm has small amounts of vitamins and minerals, but mostly starch.

Before milling equipment existed, people used stones to grind wheat into flour. Bakers separated the bran and germ from the endosperm to make white flour. People like the soft, light taste of white bread. But refining flour is a long, hard job. White flour used to be expensive. Only wealthy people could afford it.

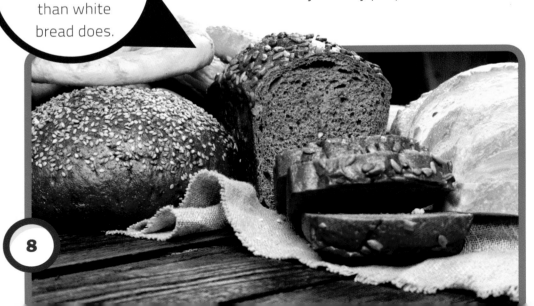

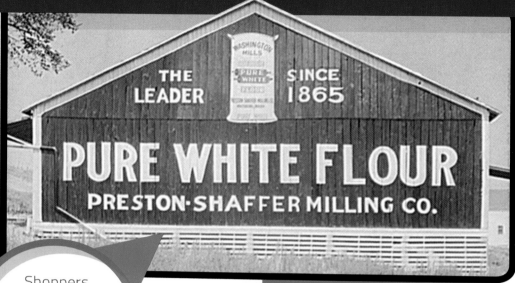

Shoppers demanded white flour once mills made it more affordable.

Poor people ate brown bread made from whole-grain flour. Eating white bread became a sign of wealth.

When milling machinery came into use, white bread became cheap. More people started to eat it. It became a staple for many people who could not afford more expensive meats and produce. Two diseases, beriberi and pellagra, became common. Researchers found the cause was a lack of B vitamins. Governments passed new laws. They required flour makers to add iron and B vitamins back into white flour.

23
Percent increase in whole grain consumption since 2008.

- The wheat grain's bran and germ are removed to make white flour.
- White flour is enriched to replace lost nutrients.
- Whole-grain bread is more nutritious.

Whole-grain bread is healthier than white bread. It has all of the wheat's fiber and nutrients. To know whether bread is whole wheat or whole grain, look at the label. Whole-grain flour will be an ingredient. Sometimes brown bread is just white bread with added brown coloring.

9

Busted: Eating Fat Makes You Fat

In the 1980s, health experts observed a rise in the number of overweight Americans. The experts believed a high-fat diet was the cause. They recommended Americans cut fat calories to less than 30 percent of daily intake. This started a low-fat craze in food products. The craze continued into the following decades.

To meet the new low-fat guidelines, food makers removed the fat from processed foods. But removing the fat also removed flavor. To make the foods tasty, companies replaced the fat with sugar. But the body converts sugar into energy. Any leftover energy is stored as fat. Many people believed these low-fat

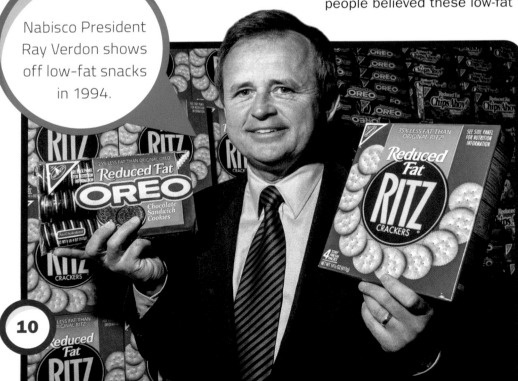

Nabisco President Ray Verdon shows off low-fat snacks in 1994.

9

Calories in 1 gram of fat.

- Experts blamed high-fat diets for weight gain in the 1980s.
- Food producers replaced fat with sugar.
- People continued to gain weight because they continued to eat the same amount of calories.

Staying active will help you maintain a healthy weight.

foods were healthy. But today, more than two-thirds of adults are still overweight or obese. So are nearly 32 percent of children.

Research in the last 35 years found the calorie is an important factor in healthy weight control. A calorie is the unit of energy that foods produce in the body. When you eat, you take in calories. When you exercise, you burn calories. Consuming more calories than you burn results in weight gain. Burning more calories than you eat results in weight loss. Avoiding fat will not keep you from gaining weight if you are still taking in more calories than you burn.

Eating fat will not make you fat unless you eat more calories than you burn.

TRANS FAT

In the early 1920s, food makers discovered how to turn liquid vegetable oil into solid margarine and shortening. These trans fats became popular replacements for saturated fats such as butter. In time, evidence linked trans fat to an increased risk of several diseases. Today, nutrition experts advise people to avoid trans fat.

11

Busted: All Carbohydrates Are the Same

During the low-fat craze of the 1990s, people avoided eating fatty foods. Instead, they ate more carbohydrates such as bread, pasta, and rice. Despite the change in diet, the average American was overweight. In 1992, Dr. Robert Atkins, a cardiologist, wrote a bestselling book. His advice was to avoid all carbohydrates. Instead, he urged people to eat foods high in fat and protein. Many people switched from a low-fat to a

low-carbohydrate diet. Food makers began to make "low-carb" foods.

In the mid-1800s, a French scientist Claude Bernard discovered how the human body converts carbohydrates and fat to energy. Plants make carbohydrates when they turn sunlight into energy. They store the carbohydrates as sugar, or glucose. The plant needs glucose to grow. When people eat plant foods, this process is reversed. Digesting plant carbohydrates converts them back into energy.

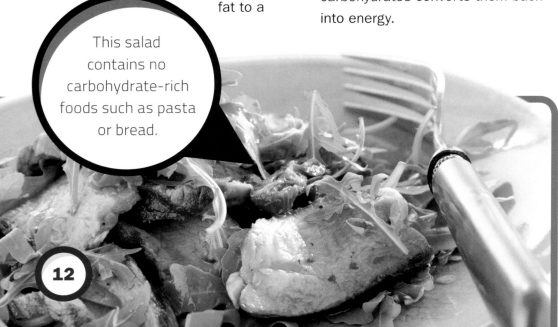

This salad contains no carbohydrate-rich foods such as pasta or bread.

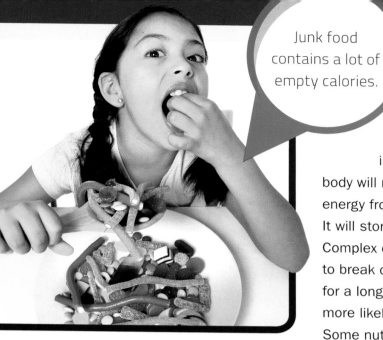

There are two kinds of carbohydrates. Simple carbohydrates are found in fruits, milk, and vegetables. In their natural states, these foods also contain important nutrients. But when simple carbohydrates are separated from foods, they become sugars. These sugars are empty calories. They lack vitamins, minerals, and fiber. Complex carbohydrates are found in whole grains, beans, starchy vegetables, nuts, and seeds. They are loaded with fiber, vitamins, and minerals.

When people eat simple or complex carbohydrates, their bodies break them down. First, the carbohydrates become sugars and finally

energy. Simple carbohydrates are easily broken down into energy. Often, the body will not be able to use all the energy from simple carbohydrates. It will store the extra energy as fat. Complex carbohydrates take longer to break down. They provide energy for a longer period. The body is more likely to use all the energy. Some nutritionists believe the Atkins diet unnecessarily restricts all carbohydrates. Not all carbohydrates cause humans to gain weight. Complex carbohydrates provide just enough energy for the body to use.

4
Grams of sugar in 1 teaspoon of sugar.

- Simple carbohydrates are easily broken down into energy.
- Complex carbohydrates take longer for the body to digest.
- Simple carbohydrates are more easily stored as fat.

Busted: Eggs Cause Heart Disease

Eggs are nutritious foods full of protein and nutrients. In 1961, the American Heart Association linked eating eggs to heart disease. In 1990, the United States dietary guidelines recommended people limit eating eggs. Egg yolks are high in cholesterol. Scientists believed eating egg yolks would raise blood cholesterol levels in humans. High blood cholesterol is linked to heart disease. The guidelines encouraged people to avoid eating egg yolks. Food companies developed egg alternatives and low-cholesterol products.

In the early 1900s, a Russian researcher experimented with rabbits and found evidence that eating cholesterol was harmful. In the 1940s, US researchers thought they also found a link between dietary cholesterol and heart disease. This research led to the

BROWN EGGS

Chicken eggs can be white, brown, blue, or green. Some people think brown eggs are healthier. But all fresh eggs are equally good for you. The color of the eggshell depends on the breed of chicken that laid it.

25
Years eggs were considered bad for your heart.

- Eggs are high in protein, vitamin D, and other nutrients.
- In 1961, experts linked eating eggs to heart disease.
- Years later, experts found eggs do not put healthy people at risk for heart disease.

US government issuing its dietary guidelines on eggs.

But further studies show cholesterol itself is not harmful. Blood cholesterol levels are determined by two types of cholesterol. Low-density lipoprotein, or LDL, cholesterol is bad cholesterol. It produces a thick hard substance that clogs arteries. High-density lipoprotein, or HDL, cholesterol is good cholesterol. It carries the LDL cholesterol away from the arteries. Having too much LDL

cholesterol and too little HDL cholesterol contributes to heart disease.

Scientists now think the cholesterol in egg yolks does not raise blood cholesterol. For most healthy people, eating an egg every day is okay.

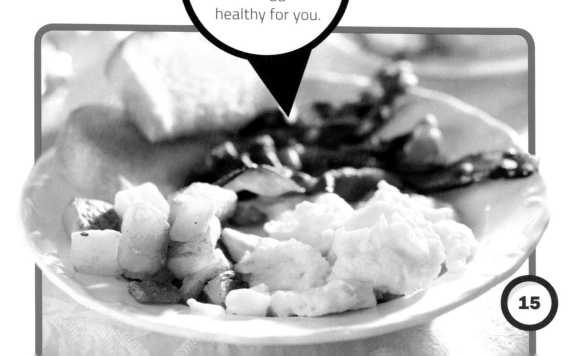

Scientists have debated whether or not eggs are healthy for you.

Busted: Everyone Needs Eight Glasses of Water Daily

In 1945, government scientists advised adults to drink 10.5 cups (2.5 L) of water a day. They acknowledged most of this water could come from foods. Fruits and vegetables have high water contents. But health experts urged adults to drink eight 8-ounce (2.5 L) glasses of water each day. They simplified the advice in the term "8 × 8." They ignored the water in other drinks and foods. Today, the 8 × 8 rule is seen in health magazines, websites, and on TV.

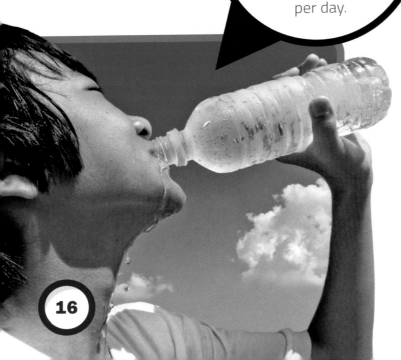

For decades, scientists have recommended Americans drink eight glasses of water per day.

Getting enough water is important. It helps the body maintain a normal temperature. It makes joints work well. It protects the spinal cord and tissues. It helps the body get rid of waste. But no scientific evidence has been found to support the 8 × 8 guideline.

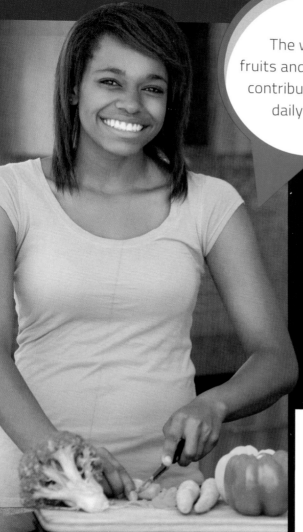

The water in fruits and vegetables contributes to your daily intake.

THINK ABOUT IT

A company that sells bottled water funded two reports. The reports found Americans do not drink enough water. Is it important to learn who pays for research? Why might a research project funded by a food company be less trustworthy than one funded by a science foundation?

Some people may need to drink more than others. They may be ill, do heavy physical work, or live in hot climates. In these cases, water is the best choice. It has no sugar, chemicals, caffeine, or calories. But healthy people who drink water when thirsty do not need to follow the 8 × 8 rule.

50 billion
Water bottles purchased each year in the United States.

- In 1945, government guidelines advised eight glasses of water per day.
- Experts failed to add that food and other drinks contain water.
- No scientific evidence supports the 8 × 8 rule.

Busted: Eating Extra Protein Makes You Stronger

Proteins are an important part of a healthy diet. They provide structure for the body's cells and tissues. They help these cells and tissues function properly. Some people worry about eating enough protein. Muscles are made of protein. People think eating extra protein will build more muscle.

Your body is 15 percent protein. Protein makes up the muscles that keep your body working. The more muscle you have, the more calories you burn, and the more food you need. Proteins are important for your cells, too. They constantly break down and rebuild your body.

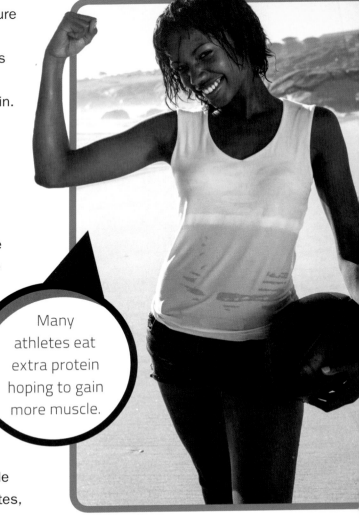

Many athletes eat extra protein hoping to gain more muscle.

In 1827, British chemist William Prout was the first to identify that foods are made of water, fat, carbohydrates, and protein. More than

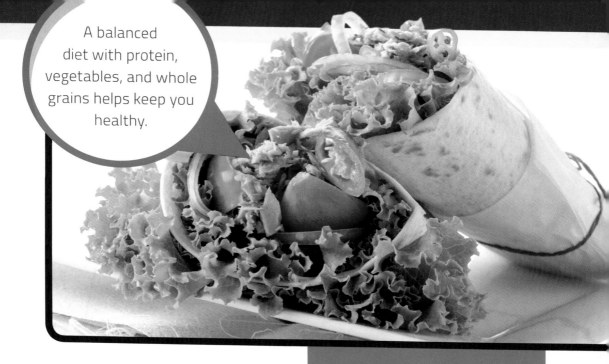

A balanced diet with protein, vegetables, and whole grains helps keep you healthy.

100 years later, in 1930, American chemist William Rose identified essential amino acids. These are the molecules that make up protein. They work together like links in a chain. Your body breaks down and rebuilds itself. It uses amino acids as building blocks. Essential amino acids are the ones your body cannot make. People should eat protein containing essential amino acids every day.

Eating animal protein or a combination of vegetable proteins will provide all the essential amino acids. Any extra over what the body needs will not create more muscle.

5
Ounces (28 g) of protein needed per day for most 9- to 17-year-olds.

- Protein is composed of amino acids.
- Vegetables and animal foods provide essential amino acids.
- Eating extra protein will not increase muscle mass.

Healthy people who eat a variety of whole, unrefined foods, get plenty of protein. But protein does not cause muscle growth. Gaining muscle is a result of exercise, not food intake.

Busted: Multivitamins Make You Healthier

Two American chemists, Max Tishler and Robert Williams, discovered a way to make synthetic vitamins in 1933 and 1940. In 1941, the US government published the first Recommended Dietary Allowances (RDAs). The guidelines gave suggestions for vitamins, minerals, protein, and energy.

Soon, companies were making multivitamin pills with the RDAs of vitamins and minerals. Today, more than one-half of Americans take a daily multivitamin supplement. Multivitamin sales in the United States totaled an estimated $36.7 billion in 2014.

Millions of Americans take a daily multivitamin.

FAT- AND WATER-SOLUBLE VITAMINS

B vitamins and vitamin C are contained in the watery parts of food. Blood absorbs them when food is digested. Extra water-soluble vitamins are excreted in your urine. Fat-soluble vitamins do not go into the bloodstream. These include vitamins A, D, E, and K. They are processed in the stomach and small intestine. Then, they are stored in the liver and fat tissue for later use.

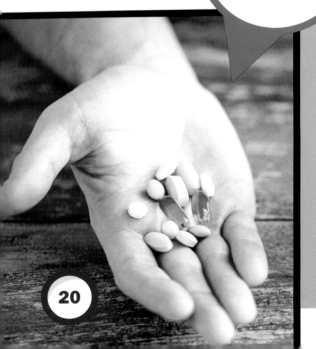

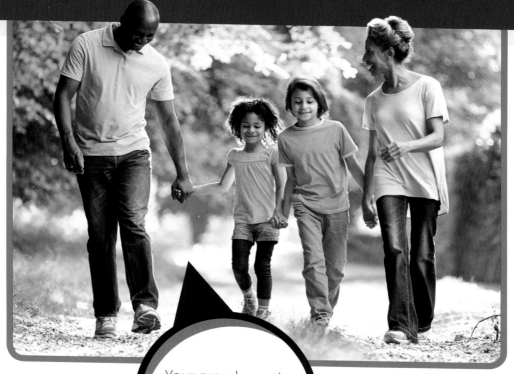

Your grandparents may need to take a multivitamin, but you may not.

Scientists know vitamins and minerals from food are linked to good health. A balanced diet is all someone needs to meet their RDAs. But vitamin pills are useful in some cases. They can cure diseases caused by nutritional deficiencies. Pregnant women, the elderly, vegans, and people with certain diseases can benefit, too. But taking more vitamins in supplements has not been linked to improved health. Megadoses of some vitamins, especially fat-soluble ones, can even be harmful.

600

International units of vitamin D a 9- to 13-year-old should get every day.

- Scientific research shows people who eat a balanced diet do not benefit further from a multivitamin pill.
- Vitamins can be harmful in megadoses.
- People who are malnourished, ill, or have special needs may benefit from supplements.

Busted: Eating Superfoods Will Keep You Healthy

Media sources often report that certain foods are super because they prevent disease. They claim others add years to your life. Broccoli can undo damage from diabetes. Eating dark chocolate can cut the risk of stroke. A daily dose of garlic can save your life. Blueberries improve your memory. Eating fish makes you smarter. But will eating these foods guarantee a healthy and long life?

The term *superfoods* became popular in the 1990s. It was introduced in a cookbook. The authors advised people to eat whole plant foods for better health. Nutrition writers adopted the term. They continue to publish reports about superfoods. Specific foods such as kale, oranges, yogurt, and salmon became super. Unusual foods such as

acai berries and chia seeds were supposedly miraculously healthy.

There is no official definition of a superfood. But foods high in antioxidants are usually singled out. Antioxidants fight chemicals in our

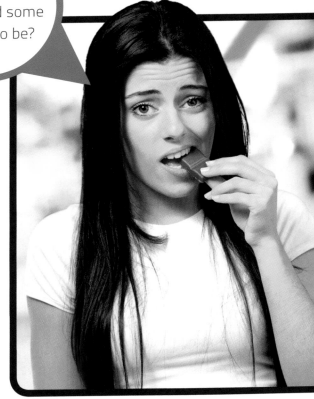

Is chocolate the superfood some claim it to be?

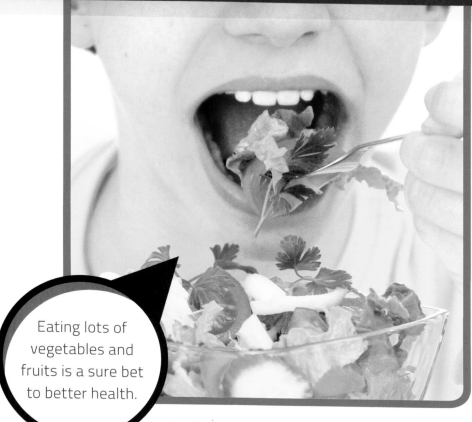

Eating lots of vegetables and fruits is a sure bet to better health.

bodies that can cause damage. Vitamins C and E, beta-carotene, and some minerals act as antioxidants.

Many food companies selling products with antioxidants claimed their foods were super. But scientific evidence since 1990 has not shown that antioxidants alone prevent disease. Eating any single food cannot guarantee a healthy, long life. Science says eating a variety of whole plant foods is the best way to stay healthy and live longer.

4
Minimum number of daily cups of fruits and vegetables recommended for 9- to 13-year-olds.

- The term *superfood* is often used for foods high in antioxidants.
- Antioxidants fight chemicals that cause disease.
- No single superfood can guarantee good health or a long life.

Busted: Sugar Makes You Hyper

Parents often accuse their kids of fidgeting after eating too much cake or candy. Schools have rules restricting sweets. Teachers do not want their students to lose concentration during the school day. Why do so many people believe sugar makes children behave badly?

In 1973, allergist Benjamin Feingold developed a popular diet. He claimed eliminating artificial additives, such as dyes and chemical flavors, could prevent behavior problems in children. Sugar was considered an additive. Scientists began to study the connection between diet and behavior.

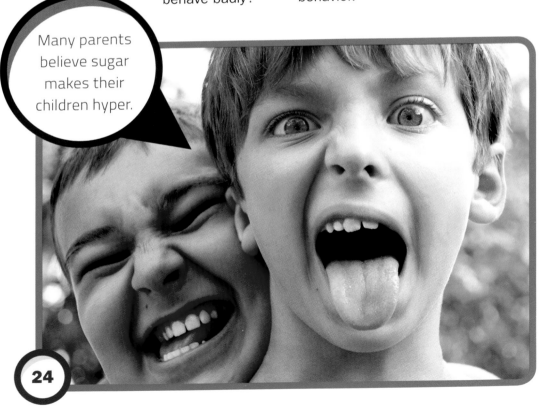

Many parents believe sugar makes their children hyper.

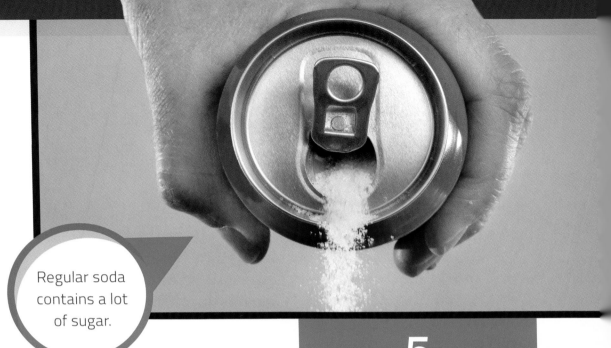

Regular soda contains a lot of sugar.

Studies conducted since then have failed to link dietary sugar and hyperactivity. But the myth persists. Kids eat sugary foods at birthday or holiday parties. Behaviorists think parents and teachers mistake the cause of kids' hyper behaviors. It may be the event that is causing the change in behavior, not the sugar.

There are plenty of good reasons to limit sugar intake. Sugar has no nutrients but lots of calories. It might replace healthier foods in your diet. Too many calories can lead to weight gain. Sugar can also cause tooth decay. But sugar is not the cause of hyperactivity.

5

Approximate teaspoons of sugar in a 12-ounce (355 mL) can of sweetened soda.

- Many parents and teachers blame sugar consumption for children's behavioral problems.
- No link has been found between eating sweets and becoming overactive.
- Sugar should be limited because it contains empty calories and causes tooth decay.

Busted: Fresh Fruits and Veggies Are Best

Government guidelines tell people to eat more fresh produce. Scientific evidence links eating fruits and vegetables to good health. Fresh produce is more available in grocery stores and farmers' markets than ever before. Packaged produce that is already washed and cut is quick for people to prepare.

After it is picked, produce begins to lose its nutrients to heat, light, and oxygen. Refrigeration slows but does not stop the loss. Slicing or cutting also increases the loss of nutrients. The longer produce sits in the store or kitchen, the fewer nutrients they contain.

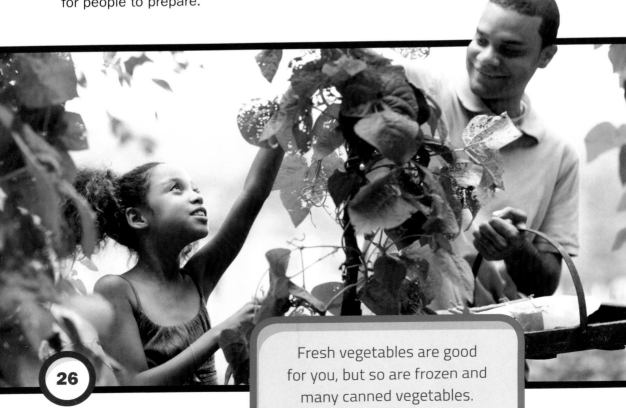

Fresh vegetables are good for you, but so are frozen and many canned vegetables.

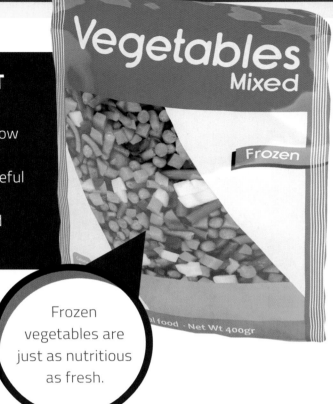

THINK ABOUT IT

The US Food and Drug Administration regulates how food manufacturers label their products. Why is it useful to understand how to read the nutrition labels on food packaging?

Frozen food is processed right after it is picked. It cannot spoil. A 2013 study compared fresh and frozen fruits and vegetables. Researchers analyzed the vitamins and minerals in both. They found fresh and frozen foods were equally nutritious. But after five days, the fresh foods lost vitamins. The frozen foods kept their nutrients.

What about canned fruits and vegetables? Canning sometimes lowers the amount of nutrients and adds sodium. But it still has the same nutrients as days-old fresh produce. It has the same nutrients as cooked frozen produce, too. Cooking reduces the nutrient levels of all produce.

Frozen vegetables are just as nutritious as fresh.

1917
Year Clarence Birdseye invented flash-frozen food.

- Most fresh fruits and vegetables lose nutrients if they sit too long before being eaten.
- Frozen and canned foods are preserved immediately.
- Frozen and canned foods are good alternatives to fresh.

27

Fact Sheet

- The human body needs a variety of vitamins to function properly. Vitamin A supports your immune system, bones, and vision. Your body uses vitamin C to make and repair organs and tissues. B vitamins help your body get or make energy from food.

- All whole foods keep you healthy, but no single food has super powers. Chocolate, coffee, berries, and broccoli are often called superfoods. But none of these foods alone will keep you healthy. Add them to a diet rich in vegetables, fruits, lean protein, and complex carbohydrates.

- Bread with 100 percent whole grain has more fiber and nutrients than white bread. Eggs are a good source of protein and are not linked to heart disease. Frozen and canned produce can be as nutritious as fresh.

- Eating a well-balanced diet will provide your body with plenty of protein. Eating a wide variety of whole foods will give you the vitamins you need. Healthy carbohydrates are an important part of a balanced diet.

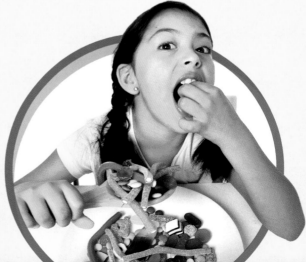

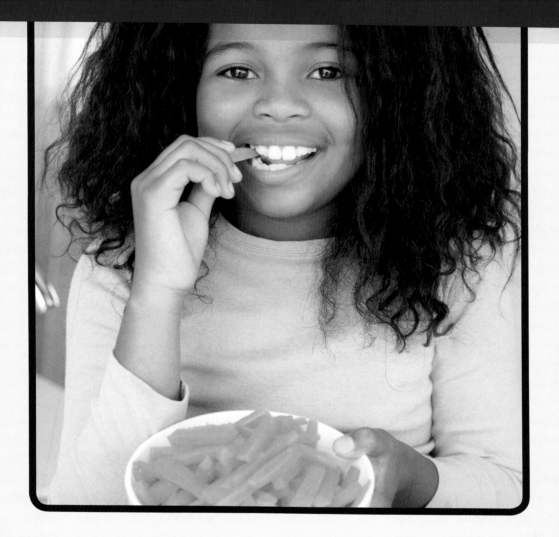

- Many processed foods have added sugars. Some added sugars are natural, but others, such as high fructose corn syrup, are created in a lab. Americans eat much more sugar than doctors recommend. The average American eats about 20 teaspoons of sugar per day. But teens should get fewer than 9 teaspoons of sugar per day.

- To maintain a healthy weight, balance your calorie intake and output. Do not eat too much sugar, which contains empty calories. Water is a better beverage choice than sweetened beverages.

Glossary

digest
To break food down into energy in the body.

energy
Power to do work or be active.

fiber
The indigestible part of plants that helps the body digest other food.

glucose
Sugar found in plants that is the source of energy for all living things.

mineral
A solid chemical the body needs to function properly.

nutrients
Substances the body needs to function properly.

produce
Fresh vegetables and fruits.

protein
Substance needed for life, composed of a chain of amino acids.

radar
Device that locates objects using radio waves.

saturated fat
Fat that is solid at room temperature.

vitamins
Substances needed in small amounts to help the body develop.

For More Information

Books

Pollan, Michael. *The Omnivore's Dilemma: Young Readers Edition.* New York: Dial Books, 2009.

Schrier, Allyson Valentine. *Eat Right: Your Guide to Maintaining a Healthy Diet.* Mankato, MN: Capstone, 2012.

Ventura, Marne. *The 12 Biggest Breakthroughs in Food Technology.* North Mankato, MN: Peterson Publishing Company, 2015.

Visit 12StoryLibrary.com

Scan the code or use your school's login at **12StoryLibrary.com** for recent updates about this topic and a full digital version of this book. Enjoy free access to:

- Digital ebook
- Breaking news updates
- Live content feeds
- Videos, interactive maps, and graphics
- Additional web resources

Note to educators: Visit 12StoryLibrary.com/register to sign up for free premium website access. Enjoy live content plus a full digital version of every 12-Story Library book you own for every student at your school.

Index

About the Author

Marne Ventura writes fiction and nonfiction for children. A former elementary teacher, she also contributes stories and articles to children's magazines. Marne lives with her husband on the central coast of California.

READ MORE FROM 12-STORY LIBRARY

Every 12-Story Library book is available in many formats. For more information, visit 12StoryLibrary.com.